DR. BARBARA'S CURE FOR EPILEPSY

Simple guide to Harnessing the power of natural and herbal to heal and cure epilepsy for your optimal well-being

Odesa Mulan

Table of Contents

COPYRIGHT © 2023

CHAPTER ONE

Understanding Epilepsy: Causes, Types, and Symptoms

Epilepsy is a neurological disorder characterized by recurrent, unprovoked seizures. It affects people of all ages and can have a significant impact on their quality of life. Understanding the causes, types, and symptoms of epilepsy is crucial for proper diagnosis, treatment, and management of the condition.

Causes of Epilepsy:

The exact cause of epilepsy can vary from person to person. In some cases, there may be a clear identifiable cause, while in others, the cause may be unknown. Common causes of epilepsy include:

1. **Genetic Factors:** Genetics play a significant role in the development of epilepsy. Individuals with a family history of the condition are at a higher risk of developing epilepsy themselves. Certain genetic mutations or abnormalities can increase susceptibility to seizures.

2. **Brain Injuries:** Traumatic brain injuries resulting from accidents, falls, or other traumatic events can lead to epilepsy. These injuries disrupt normal brain function and increase the likelihood of seizures occurring.

3. **Brain Tumors:** Tumors in the brain can interfere with normal brain activity and trigger seizures. The location and size of the tumor can impact the type and frequency of seizures experienced by the individual.

4. **Infections:** Certain infections of the brain, such as meningitis, encephalitis, or brain abscesses, can cause inflammation and damage to brain tissue, leading to epilepsy. Infections that affect the central nervous system can increase the risk of seizures.

5. **Developmental Disorders:** Some developmental disorders, such as autism spectrum disorder or neurofibromatosis, are associated with an increased risk of epilepsy. These disorders can affect brain development and increase susceptibility to seizures.

6. **Stroke:** Strokes can cause damage to brain tissue due to interrupted blood flow, leading to epilepsy. The risk of developing epilepsy after a stroke depends on the severity and location of the brain damage.

7. **Metabolic Disorders:** Certain metabolic disorders, such as diabetes or electrolyte imbalances, can disrupt normal brain function and trigger seizures. Metabolic abnormalities can affect the electrical activity of the brain, leading to epileptic seizures.

8. **Drug and Alcohol Abuse:** Substance abuse, including drugs and alcohol, can increase the risk of epilepsy. Prolonged substance abuse can lead to changes in brain chemistry and structure, making seizures more likely to occur.

It's important to note that in many cases, the exact cause of epilepsy may not be identified, and it may be classified as "idiopathic epilepsy."

Types of Epilepsy:

Epilepsy is not a single disorder but rather a spectrum of conditions characterized by recurrent seizures. There are many different types of epilepsy, each with its own unique characteristics and seizure patterns. Some of the most common types of epilepsy include:

1. **Generalized Epilepsy:** Generalized epilepsy involves seizures that affect both sides of the brain simultaneously. These seizures typically involve loss of consciousness and may cause convulsions or muscle stiffening. Types of generalized epilepsy include:

   - Absence Seizures: Characterized by brief episodes of staring and unconsciousness.

   - Tonic-Clonic Seizures: Also known as grand mal seizures, these seizures involve loss of consciousness, muscle rigidity, and convulsions.

- Myoclonic Seizures: Characterized by sudden, brief muscle jerks or twitches.

- Atonic Seizures: Also known as drop attacks, these seizures cause sudden loss of muscle tone, leading to falls or collapses.

2. **Focal (Partial) Epilepsy:** Focal epilepsy involves seizures that originate in a specific area of the brain. These seizures may or may not involve loss of consciousness, depending on the area of the brain affected. Types of focal epilepsy include:

   - Simple Partial Seizures: Seizures that do not impair consciousness and may cause sensory or motor symptoms.

   - Complex Partial Seizures: Seizures that impair consciousness and may cause confusion, automatisms (repetitive movements), or unusual behaviors.

   - Focal Aware Seizures: Seizures that do not impair consciousness and the individual remains aware of their surroundings.

   - Focal Impaired Awareness Seizures: Seizures that impair consciousness and the individual may appear dazed or confused.

3. **Epileptic Syndromes:** Some types of epilepsy are classified as syndromes, which are characterized by specific clinical

features and seizure patterns. Examples of epileptic syndromes include:

- Lennox-Gastaut Syndrome: Characterized by multiple seizure types, intellectual disability, and abnormal EEG patterns.

- Dravet Syndrome: A severe form of epilepsy that begins in infancy and is associated with developmental delays and frequent seizures.

- West Syndrome: Characterized by infantile spasms, developmental regression, and abnormal EEG patterns.

Symptoms of Epilepsy:

The symptoms of epilepsy can vary widely depending on the type of seizure and the area of the brain affected. Common symptoms of epilepsy may include:

1. **Seizures:** The hallmark symptom of epilepsy is recurrent seizures. Seizures can manifest in various ways, including:

   - Convulsions or muscle stiffening (tonic-clonic seizures)

   - Brief episodes of staring and unconsciousness (absence seizures)

   - Sudden, brief muscle jerks or twitches (myoclonic seizures)

- Sudden loss of muscle tone, leading to falls or collapses (atonic seizures)

- Sensory or motor symptoms, such as tingling, numbness, or weakness (simple partial seizures)

2. **Aura:** Some individuals with epilepsy may experience an aura or warning sign before a seizure occurs. Auras can manifest as visual disturbances, strange smells or tastes, or feelings of déjà vu or fear.

3. **Loss of Consciousness:** Many types of seizures involve loss of consciousness, during which the individual may appear dazed, confused, or unresponsive.

4. **Automatisms:** Complex partial seizures may involve automatisms, which are repetitive, purposeless movements such as lip smacking, chewing, or fidgeting.

5. **Postictal Symptoms:** After a seizure, individuals may experience postictal symptoms, including confusion, fatigue, headache, or muscle soreness.

It's essential to recognize the signs and symptoms of epilepsy and seek medical attention if you or someone you know experiences recurrent seizures or any other concerning symptoms.

In conclusion, epilepsy is a complex neurological disorder characterized by recurrent seizures. While the exact cause of epilepsy can vary, common factors include genetic predisposition, brain injuries, tumors, infections, and metabolic disorders. Epilepsy encompasses various types of seizures, including generalized and focal seizures, as well as specific epileptic syndromes. Recognizing the symptoms of epilepsy and understanding its causes and types are crucial for proper diagnosis, treatment, and management of the condition.

CHAPTER TWO

Herbal Medicine as a Complementary Approach to Epilepsy Treatment

Epilepsy is a neurological disorder characterized by recurrent seizures, affecting millions of people worldwide. While conventional medical treatments such as antiepileptic drugs (AEDs) are the primary approach to managing epilepsy, there is growing interest in complementary and alternative therapies, including herbal medicine. Herbal medicine, also known as botanical medicine or phytotherapy, involves the use of plant-derived substances to prevent or treat various medical conditions. In the context of epilepsy, herbal medicine is often explored as a complementary approach to conventional treatment strategies. This article delves into the potential benefits, safety considerations, and common herbal remedies used in the management of epilepsy.

Potential Benefits of Herbal Medicine in Epilepsy Treatment:

1. **Anticonvulsant Properties:** Many herbs possess compounds with anticonvulsant properties, meaning they have the potential to reduce the frequency and severity of seizures. These compounds may act through various mechanisms, such as modulating neurotransmitter activity, reducing

neuronal excitability, or enhancing inhibitory pathways in the brain.

2. **Neuroprotective Effects:** Some herbal remedies exhibit neuroprotective effects, which can help prevent or minimize neuronal damage associated with seizures. Neuroprotective compounds found in certain herbs may protect against oxidative stress, inflammation, and excitotoxicity, thereby preserving normal brain function and reducing seizure susceptibility.

3. **Anxiolytic and Antidepressant Effects:** Epilepsy is often associated with comorbid psychiatric conditions such as anxiety and depression. Certain herbal remedies have anxiolytic (anxiety-reducing) and antidepressant properties, which can help improve mood, reduce stress, and enhance overall well-being in individuals with epilepsy.

4. **Improved Quality of Life:** Herbal medicine may contribute to an improved quality of life for individuals with epilepsy by alleviating seizure-related symptoms, reducing medication side effects, and promoting overall health and vitality. Integrating herbal remedies into a comprehensive treatment plan can offer holistic support for physical, emotional, and psychological well-being.

Safety Considerations for Herbal Medicine Use in Epilepsy:

While herbal medicine holds promise as a complementary approach to epilepsy treatment, it is essential to exercise caution and be aware of potential safety considerations:

1. **Drug Interactions:** Some herbs may interact with antiepileptic drugs (AEDs) or other medications, altering their effectiveness or causing adverse effects. Individuals taking AEDs should consult with a healthcare professional before incorporating herbal remedies into their treatment regimen to minimize the risk of drug interactions.

2. **Quality and Purity:** The quality and purity of herbal products can vary widely, and contamination or adulteration with toxic substances may pose health risks. It is advisable to choose herbal remedies from reputable sources that adhere to quality standards and undergo rigorous testing for safety and efficacy.

3. **Allergic Reactions:** Allergic reactions to certain herbs are possible, especially in individuals with sensitivities or allergies to specific plants or botanicals. It is important to be cautious when trying new herbal remedies and discontinue use if any adverse reactions occur.

4. **Dosage and Administration:** Herbal remedies should be used with caution, and dosage recommendations should be

followed carefully to avoid toxicity or adverse effects. Herbal preparations vary in potency, and excessive consumption may lead to unintended consequences.

5. **Pregnancy and Lactation:** Pregnant or breastfeeding individuals should exercise caution when using herbal remedies, as some herbs may pose risks to fetal development or infant health. It is advisable to consult with a healthcare provider before using herbal medicine during pregnancy or lactation.

Common Herbal Remedies for Epilepsy:

Several herbs have been traditionally used in the management of epilepsy, although scientific evidence supporting their efficacy is limited. Some common herbal remedies explored for epilepsy treatment include:

1. **Valerian (Valeriana officinalis):** Valerian root is traditionally used as a sedative and anticonvulsant agent. It may help reduce anxiety, promote relaxation, and improve sleep quality in individuals with epilepsy.

2. **Passionflower (Passiflora incarnata):** Passionflower has anxiolytic and sedative properties, which may help alleviate anxiety and promote relaxation. It is sometimes used as a complementary therapy for epilepsy to reduce stress and nervous tension.

3. **Lavender (Lavandula angustifolia):** Lavender oil is known for its calming and mood-stabilizing effects. Inhalation or topical application of lavender essential oil may help reduce anxiety and stress levels in individuals with epilepsy.

4. **Ginkgo (Ginkgo biloba):** Ginkgo extract is thought to improve cerebral blood flow and exert neuroprotective effects. While research on ginkgo for epilepsy is limited, some studies suggest potential benefits in reducing seizure frequency and improving cognitive function.

5. **Cannabidiol (CBD):** CBD is a non-psychoactive cannabinoid derived from the cannabis plant. It has gained attention for its potential anticonvulsant properties and is currently being investigated as a treatment for certain forms of epilepsy, such as Dravet syndrome and Lennox-Gastaut syndrome.

Conclusion:

Herbal medicine offers a diverse array of plant-derived remedies that may hold potential as complementary approaches to epilepsy treatment. While some herbs exhibit anticonvulsant, neuroprotective, and anxiolytic properties, scientific evidence supporting their efficacy and safety in epilepsy is limited. It is crucial for individuals with epilepsy to consult with healthcare professionals before integrating herbal remedies into their treatment regimen, especially considering potential drug interactions, safety considerations, and variability in product quality. Further research is needed to elucidate the mechanisms of action, optimal dosing, and long-term effects of herbal medicine in the management of epilepsy. By combining conventional medical therapies with evidence-based herbal interventions, individuals with epilepsy can access a comprehensive and personalized approach to seizure management and overall well-being.

CHAPTER THREE

Safety Precautions and Consultation Before Starting Herbal Therapy

While herbal therapy offers potential benefits for various health conditions, including epilepsy, it's essential to approach it with caution and careful consideration. Before starting any herbal treatment regimen, individuals should be aware of safety precautions and the importance of consulting with healthcare professionals. This article highlights key safety considerations and emphasizes the importance of seeking expert guidance before incorporating herbal therapy into one's healthcare routine.

Understanding Safety Precautions for Herbal Therapy:

1. **Consultation with Healthcare Professionals:** Before starting herbal therapy, individuals should consult with healthcare professionals, such as physicians, pharmacists, or herbalists. These experts can provide personalized advice based on the individual's medical history, current health status, and any medications they may be taking.

2. **Disclosure of Medical History:** Individuals should disclose their complete medical history, including any underlying health conditions, allergies, or previous adverse reactions to medications or herbal remedies. This information enables

healthcare professionals to assess potential risks and tailor treatment recommendations accordingly.

3. **Awareness of Drug Interactions:** Herbal remedies can interact with prescription medications, over-the-counter drugs, or other herbal supplements, leading to adverse effects or reduced efficacy. It's crucial to inform healthcare providers about all medications and supplements being taken to identify potential interactions and minimize risks.

4. **Quality and Purity of Herbal Products:** The quality and purity of herbal products can vary significantly among brands and manufacturers. To ensure safety and efficacy, individuals should choose herbal supplements from reputable sources that adhere to quality standards and undergo rigorous testing for purity, potency, and contaminants.

5. **Dosage and Administration Guidelines:** Herbal remedies should be used according to recommended dosage and administration guidelines provided by healthcare professionals or product labels. Excessive consumption or incorrect administration of herbal products may increase the risk of adverse effects or toxicity.

6. **Monitoring for Adverse Reactions:** Individuals should monitor themselves for any adverse reactions or side effects associated with herbal therapy. Common signs of adverse reactions may include allergic reactions, gastrointestinal

disturbances, changes in mood or behavior, or worsening of existing health conditions. If any adverse effects occur, individuals should discontinue use and seek medical attention promptly.

Consultation Before Starting Herbal Therapy:

1. **Primary Care Physician:** Individuals with epilepsy or any other medical condition should consult with their primary care physician before starting herbal therapy. Primary care physicians can assess the individual's overall health status, review their medical history, and provide guidance on integrating herbal remedies into their treatment plan safely.

2. **Neurologist or Epileptologist:** For individuals with epilepsy, consulting with a neurologist or epileptologist is essential before considering herbal therapy. These specialists can evaluate the individual's seizure history, current treatment regimen, and potential risks and benefits of herbal remedies in the context of epilepsy management.

3. **Pharmacist:** Pharmacists play a vital role in medication management and can provide valuable insights into potential drug interactions between herbal remedies and prescription medications. Individuals can consult with pharmacists to review their medication list, discuss herbal therapy options, and ensure safe and effective use of herbal supplements.

4. **Herbalist or Naturopathic Doctor:** Consulting with a qualified herbalist or naturopathic doctor can provide individuals with specialized expertise in herbal medicine and natural therapies. These practitioners can offer personalized recommendations, herbal formulations, and lifestyle modifications to support overall health and well-being.

5. **Integration of Conventional and Herbal Therapies:** Healthcare professionals can help individuals navigate the integration of conventional medical therapies and herbal remedies effectively. By collaborating with healthcare providers, individuals can access comprehensive and holistic treatment approaches that address their unique health needs while minimizing potential risks and maximizing therapeutic benefits.

In conclusion, safety precautions and consultation with healthcare professionals are essential steps before starting herbal therapy for epilepsy or any other health condition. By following these guidelines, individuals can make informed decisions, minimize potential risks, and optimize the safety and effectiveness of herbal remedies as complementary or adjunctive treatments. With proper guidance and monitoring, herbal therapy can be integrated safely and effectively into a comprehensive healthcare regimen, supporting overall health and well-being.

CHAPTER FOUR

Day 1: Introduction to Herbal Remedies for Seizure Control

Welcome to Day 1 of our exploration into herbal remedies for seizure control. In this session, we'll provide an introduction to herbal therapy for managing seizures, covering key concepts, common herbs, and considerations for incorporating herbal remedies into your treatment regimen. Let's begin by understanding the principles behind herbal therapy and its potential role in epilepsy management.

Understanding Herbal Therapy:

Herbal therapy, also known as herbal medicine or botanical medicine, involves the use of plant-derived substances to prevent, alleviate, or treat various health conditions. This practice has been an integral part of traditional medicine systems worldwide for centuries, with plants and herbs valued for their therapeutic properties and medicinal benefits.

Herbal remedies contain bioactive compounds such as alkaloids, flavonoids, terpenes, and phenolic compounds, which exert pharmacological effects on the body. These compounds may interact with biological pathways, modulate physiological processes, and exert therapeutic effects, including anticonvulsant properties for managing seizures.

Role of Herbal Remedies in Seizure Control:

Herbal remedies have been explored as complementary or alternative therapies for managing seizures, particularly in individuals with epilepsy. While conventional treatments such as antiepileptic drugs (AEDs) remain the primary approach to seizure management, herbal therapy offers additional options for individuals seeking alternative or adjunctive treatments.

The potential benefits of herbal remedies for seizure control include:

1. **Anticonvulsant Properties:** Many herbs contain compounds with anticonvulsant properties, which can help reduce the frequency and severity of seizures. These compounds may act through various mechanisms, such as enhancing inhibitory neurotransmission, modulating ion channels, or reducing neuronal excitability.

2. **Neuroprotective Effects:** Some herbal remedies exhibit neuroprotective effects, which can help preserve normal brain function and mitigate neuronal damage associated with seizures. Neuroprotective compounds found in certain herbs may protect against oxidative stress, inflammation, and neuronal injury, thereby supporting overall brain health.

3. **Anxiolytic and Sedative Effects:** Herbal remedies with anxiolytic (anxiety-reducing) and sedative properties may help alleviate stress, anxiety, and nervous tension, which are

common triggers for seizures in individuals with epilepsy. These herbs can promote relaxation, improve sleep quality, and enhance overall well-being.

4. **Potential for Fewer Side Effects:** Herbal remedies may offer a more natural and holistic approach to seizure management, potentially minimizing the risk of adverse effects commonly associated with conventional medications. Integrating herbal therapy into a comprehensive treatment plan may help reduce medication side effects and enhance treatment tolerability.

Common Herbs for Seizure Control:

Several herbs have been traditionally used for managing seizures and supporting overall brain health. While scientific evidence supporting their efficacy is limited, these herbs have gained popularity as complementary or alternative treatments for epilepsy. Some common herbs explored for seizure control include:

1. **Valerian (Valeriana officinalis):** Valerian root is known for its calming and sedative effects, making it a popular herbal remedy for anxiety, insomnia, and nervous disorders. It may help reduce seizure frequency and promote relaxation in individuals with epilepsy.

2. **Passionflower (Passiflora incarnata):** Passionflower has anxiolytic and sedative properties, which can help reduce

stress, anxiety, and nervous tension. It may be beneficial for individuals with epilepsy who experience seizures triggered by emotional stress or anxiety.

3. **Skullcap (Scutellarialateriflora):** Skullcap is traditionally used as a nervine tonic and antispasmodic agent, making it a potential herbal remedy for managing seizures and nervous system disorders. It may help calm the mind, reduce muscle spasms, and promote relaxation.

4. **Lemon Balm (Melissa officinalis):** Lemon balm is known for its calming and mood-stabilizing effects, which may help alleviate anxiety, stress, and restlessness. It may be beneficial for individuals with epilepsy who experience seizures triggered by emotional or psychological factors.

5. **Chamomile (Matricaria chamomilla):** Chamomile is prized for its calming and anti-inflammatory properties, making it a popular herbal remedy for promoting relaxation and reducing stress. It may help support overall nervous system health and alleviate seizure-related symptoms.

Conclusion:

Herbal therapy offers a diverse array of plant-derived remedies that may hold potential for managing seizures and supporting overall brain health. While scientific evidence supporting the efficacy of herbal remedies in epilepsy is limited, these natural interventions have gained recognition as complementary or alternative treatments for individuals seeking holistic approaches to seizure control. In the following sessions, we'll delve deeper into specific herbs, their mechanisms of action, and practical considerations for incorporating herbal therapy into your epilepsy management plan. Stay tuned for more insights and guidance on herbal remedies for seizure control.

CHAPTER FIVE

Day 2: Herbal Teas and Decoctions for Epilepsy Management

Welcome back to our exploration of herbal remedies for epilepsy management. In today's session, we'll delve into the world of herbal teas and decoctions, discussing their potential benefits, common ingredients, and practical considerations for incorporating them into your daily routine. Let's explore how herbal teas and decoctions can serve as soothing and therapeutic beverages for supporting overall well-being in individuals with epilepsy.

Understanding Herbal Teas and Decoctions:

Herbal teas and decoctions are liquid preparations made from various plant parts, including leaves, flowers, roots, bark, and seeds. These preparations are created by steeping or boiling herbs in water, extracting their bioactive compounds, flavors, and medicinal properties. Herbal teas and decoctions are popular beverages enjoyed for their taste, aroma, and potential health benefits.

Benefits of Herbal Teas and Decoctions for Epilepsy Management:

1. **Relaxation and Stress Reduction:** Herbal teas and decoctions containing anxiolytic and sedative herbs can help promote relaxation, reduce stress, and alleviate anxiety,

which are common triggers for seizures in individuals with epilepsy. Enjoying a warm cup of herbal tea can create a calming ritual and support emotional well-being.

2. **Hydration and Fluid Balance:** Staying hydrated is essential for maintaining overall health and supporting optimal brain function. Herbal teas and decoctions provide a hydrating and refreshing alternative to plain water, helping maintain fluid balance and supporting physiological processes in the body, including neurotransmission and detoxification.

3. **Antioxidant and Neuroprotective Effects:** Many herbs used in herbal teas and decoctions exhibit antioxidant and neuroprotective properties, which can help protect against oxidative stress, inflammation, and neuronal damage associated with seizures. Regular consumption of antioxidant-rich herbal beverages may support brain health and reduce seizure susceptibility.

4. **Digestive Support:** Some herbal teas and decoctions contain herbs with digestive-supportive properties, such as soothing the gastrointestinal tract, relieving indigestion, and promoting bowel regularity. Digestive health is closely linked to overall well-being, and herbal beverages can contribute to a healthy digestive system.

5. **Herbal Synergy and Holistic Support:** Herbal teas and decoctions often contain a blend of herbs, each contributing

its unique therapeutic properties and synergistic effects. This holistic approach to herbal therapy addresses multiple aspects of health and well-being, supporting the body's natural healing processes and promoting balance.

Common Ingredients in Herbal Teas and Decoctions for Epilepsy:

1. **Chamomile (Matricaria chamomilla):** Chamomile is prized for its calming and anti-inflammatory properties, making it a popular ingredient in herbal teas for promoting relaxation and reducing stress and anxiety.

2. **Lemon Balm (Melissa officinalis):** Lemon balm is known for its mood-stabilizing and antispasmodic effects, making it a soothing addition to herbal teas for individuals with epilepsy.

3. **Valerian (Valeriana officinalis):** Valerian root is a sedative herb used to promote relaxation and improve sleep quality. It may be included in herbal teas for its calming effects on the nervous system.

4. **Passionflower (Passiflora incarnata):** Passionflower has anxiolytic and sedative properties, making it a valuable ingredient in herbal teas for reducing stress and anxiety.

5. **Skullcap (Scutellarialateriflora):** Skullcap is traditionally used as a nervine tonic and antispasmodic agent, making it a

potential addition to herbal teas for managing seizures and nervous system disorders.

Practical Considerations for Enjoying Herbal Teas and Decoctions:

1. **Selection of High-Quality Herbs:** Choose high-quality herbs from reputable sources to ensure purity, potency, and safety. Organic and sustainably sourced herbs are preferred whenever possible.

2. **Preparation Methods:** Follow proper preparation methods for herbal teas and decoctions, including correct steeping or boiling times, water temperatures, and herb-to-water ratios. This ensures optimal extraction of medicinal compounds and flavors.

3. **Personalized Blends:** Experiment with creating personalized herbal tea blends tailored to your taste preferences and health goals. Combine different herbs to create synergistic effects and enhance therapeutic benefits.

4. **Moderation and Consistency:** Enjoy herbal teas and decoctions in moderation as part of a balanced diet and lifestyle. Consistent consumption may yield cumulative benefits over time, supporting overall health and well-being.

5. **Consultation with Healthcare Professionals:** Consult with healthcare professionals, including physicians, herbalists, or

naturopathic doctors, before incorporating herbal teas and decoctions into your epilepsy management plan. They can provide personalized recommendations and ensure compatibility with your current treatment regimen.

Conclusion:

Herbal teas and decoctions offer soothing and therapeutic beverages that can complement conventional treatments for epilepsy management. With their calming, hydrating, and antioxidant-rich properties, herbal beverages provide holistic support for individuals with epilepsy, promoting relaxation, stress reduction, and overall well-being. By incorporating high-quality herbs into your daily routine and following proper preparation methods, you can enjoy the benefits of herbal teas and decoctions as part of a balanced and integrative approach to seizure control. Stay tuned for more insights and practical tips on incorporating herbal remedies into your epilepsy management plan in the upcoming sessions.

CHAPTER SIX

Day 3: Incorporating Anti-Epileptic Herbs into Your Daily Routine

Welcome to Day 3 of our series on herbal remedies for epilepsy management. Today, we'll focus on practical strategies for incorporating anti-epileptic herbs into your daily routine. By integrating these herbs into your lifestyle in a mindful and consistent manner, you can harness their therapeutic benefits and support seizure control. Let's explore how you can incorporate anti-epileptic herbs seamlessly into your daily life.

Identifying Anti-Epileptic Herbs:

Before incorporating anti-epileptic herbs into your daily routine, it's essential to familiarize yourself with herbs that possess anticonvulsant properties. These herbs may help reduce the frequency and severity of seizures and support overall brain health. Some common anti-epileptic herbs include:

1. **Valerian (Valeriana officinalis):** Valerian root is known for its calming and sedative effects, making it a potential anti-epileptic herb for managing seizures and promoting relaxation.

2. **Passionflower (Passiflora incarnata):** Passionflower has anxiolytic and sedative properties, which may help reduce

stress, anxiety, and nervous tension, contributing to seizure control.

3. **Skullcap (Scutellarialateriflora):** Skullcap is traditionally used as a nervine tonic and antispasmodic agent, making it a potential anti-epileptic herb for managing seizures and nervous system disorders.

4. **Lemon Balm (Melissa officinalis):** Lemon balm exhibits mood-stabilizing and antispasmodic effects, which may contribute to seizure management and overall brain health.

5. **Ginkgo (Ginkgo biloba):** Ginkgo extract has neuroprotective properties and may help reduce seizure frequency and improve cognitive function in individuals with epilepsy.

Practical Tips for Incorporating Anti-Epileptic Herbs:

1. **Herbal Teas:** Enjoy herbal teas containing anti-epileptic herbs as part of your daily routine. Brew a soothing cup of herbal tea in the morning or evening to promote relaxation and stress reduction.

2. **Tinctures and Extracts:** Consider using herbal tinctures or liquid extracts made from anti-epileptic herbs. Add a few drops of herbal tincture to water, juice, or tea for easy consumption.

3. **Capsules and Tablets:** If you prefer a more convenient option, look for standardized herbal capsules or tablets containing anti-epileptic herbs. Follow the recommended dosage instructions provided on the product label.

4. **Cooking and Culinary Uses:** Incorporate anti-epileptic herbs into your cooking and culinary creations. Add fresh or dried herbs to soups, stews, salads, and stir-fries to infuse dishes with their medicinal properties.

5. **Aromatherapy:** Explore the use of essential oils derived from anti-epileptic herbs for aromatherapy. Diffuse calming essential oils or dilute them in carrier oils for topical application to promote relaxation and stress relief.

6. **Herbal Baths:** Create herbal baths using anti-epileptic herbs to promote relaxation and soothe the nervous system. Add dried herbs to a warm bath and soak for a calming and therapeutic experience.

7. **Mindfulness Practices:** Incorporate mindfulness practices such as meditation, deep breathing exercises, or yoga into your daily routine to complement the effects of anti-epileptic herbs. These practices can help reduce stress, promote relaxation, and support overall well-being.

Safety Considerations:

- **Consultation with Healthcare Professionals:** Before incorporating anti-epileptic herbs into your daily routine, consult with healthcare professionals, including physicians, neurologists, or herbalists. They can provide personalized recommendations based on your individual health needs and ensure compatibility with your current treatment regimen.

- **Dosage and Administration:** Follow recommended dosage and administration guidelines for anti-epileptic herbs to minimize the risk of adverse effects or toxicity. Start with a low dose and gradually increase as needed, paying attention to any changes in symptoms or side effects.

- **Monitoring and Feedback:** Monitor your response to anti-epileptic herbs closely and provide feedback to healthcare professionals. Keep track of any changes in seizure frequency, severity, or other symptoms, and report them during follow-up appointments.

Conclusion:

Incorporating anti-epileptic herbs into your daily routine can be a rewarding and empowering experience. By exploring different forms of herbal preparations and integrating them into your lifestyle mindfully, you can harness the therapeutic benefits of these herbs and support seizure control and overall well-being. Remember to consult with healthcare professionals for personalized guidance and monitor your response to herbal therapy closely. Stay tuned for more insights and practical tips on herbal remedies for epilepsy management in the upcoming sessions.

CHAPTER SEVEN

Day 4: Herbal Supplements and Tinctures for Seizure Prevention

Welcome to Day 4 of our series on herbal remedies for seizure prevention. Today, we'll focus on herbal supplements and tinctures, exploring their potential role in supporting seizure control and promoting overall brain health. Herbal supplements and tinctures offer concentrated forms of medicinal herbs, making them convenient and effective options for individuals seeking natural approaches to epilepsy management. Let's delve into the benefits, considerations, and practical tips for incorporating herbal supplements and tinctures into your seizure prevention regimen.

Understanding Herbal Supplements and Tinctures:

Herbal supplements and tinctures are concentrated forms of herbal extracts derived from medicinal plants. These preparations contain bioactive compounds extracted from various plant parts, including leaves, roots, flowers, and seeds, which exert therapeutic effects on the body. Herbal supplements are typically available in capsule or tablet form, while tinctures are liquid extracts made by steeping herbs in alcohol or glycerin.

Benefits of Herbal Supplements and Tinctures for Seizure Prevention:

1. **Concentration of Active Compounds:** Herbal supplements and tinctures provide concentrated doses of active compounds found in medicinal herbs, allowing for precise dosing and targeted therapeutic effects. This can be particularly beneficial for individuals seeking potent and effective natural remedies for seizure prevention.

2. **Convenience and Accessibility:** Herbal supplements and tinctures offer convenient and accessible options for incorporating herbal therapy into your daily routine. They can be easily taken as part of a daily supplement regimen or added to beverages for easy consumption.

3. **Customization and Personalization:** Herbal supplements and tinctures allow for customization and personalization of dosage and herbal blends, catering to individual preferences and health needs. This flexibility enables individuals to tailor their herbal therapy regimen to suit their unique requirements for seizure prevention.

4. **Bioavailability and Absorption:** Liquid herbal tinctures are readily absorbed by the body, allowing for efficient delivery of medicinal compounds into the bloodstream. This enhances bioavailability and ensures that the therapeutic

benefits of herbal remedies are maximized for seizure prevention.

Common Herbal Supplements and Tinctures for Seizure Prevention:

1. **Valerian Root Supplement:** Valerian root supplements are available in capsule or tablet form and are commonly used for promoting relaxation, reducing stress, and supporting seizure prevention.

2. **Passionflower Tincture:** Passionflower tincture is a concentrated liquid extract of passionflower, known for its anxiolytic and sedative effects. It may help reduce anxiety, calm the nervous system, and support seizure control.

3. **Skullcap Capsules:** Skullcap capsules contain powdered skullcap herb, traditionally used as a nervine tonic and antispasmodic agent. They may help manage seizures and support overall nervous system health.

4. **Lemon Balm Tincture:** Lemon balm tincture is a liquid extract made from lemon balm leaves, prized for its mood-stabilizing and antispasmodic properties. It may be beneficial for individuals with epilepsy seeking natural remedies for seizure prevention.

Practical Tips for Incorporating Herbal Supplements and Tinctures:

1. **Consultation with Healthcare Professionals:** Before starting any herbal supplements or tinctures for seizure prevention, consult with healthcare professionals, including physicians or herbalists. They can provide personalized recommendations, dosage guidance, and monitor your response to herbal therapy.

2. **Start Slowly and Monitor Effects:** Begin with a low dose of herbal supplements or tinctures and gradually increase as needed while monitoring your response closely. Pay attention to any changes in seizure frequency, severity, or other symptoms and adjust dosage accordingly.

3. **Follow Dosage Instructions:** Follow recommended dosage instructions provided on the product label or as advised by healthcare professionals. Take herbal supplements or tinctures consistently and at regular intervals to maintain therapeutic levels in the body.

4. **Consider Combination Therapy:** Explore the potential synergistic effects of combining multiple herbal supplements or tinctures for enhanced seizure prevention. Consult with healthcare professionals to determine appropriate combinations and dosages based on your individual health needs.

5. **Quality and Purity:** Choose high-quality herbal supplements and tinctures from reputable sources that adhere to stringent quality standards and undergo rigorous testing for purity, potency, and contaminants.

Conclusion:

Herbal supplements and tinctures offer concentrated forms of medicinal herbs that can support seizure prevention and promote overall brain health. By incorporating these natural remedies into your daily routine and following proper dosage and administration guidelines, you can harness the therapeutic benefits of herbal therapy for epilepsy management. Remember to consult with healthcare professionals for personalized guidance and monitor your response to herbal supplements and tinctures closely. Stay tuned for more insights and practical tips on herbal remedies for epilepsy management in the upcoming sessions.

CHAPTER EIGHT

Day 5: Stress Reduction Techniques and Herbal Support for Epilepsy

Welcome to Day 5 of our series on herbal remedies for epilepsy management. Today, we'll explore stress reduction techniques and herbal support strategies tailored specifically for individuals living with epilepsy. Stress is a common trigger for seizures in many individuals, and adopting stress management techniques alongside herbal remedies can play a crucial role in seizure prevention and overall well-being. Let's delve into effective stress reduction methods and herbal support for epilepsy.

Understanding the Impact of Stress on Epilepsy:

Stress is known to exacerbate seizure activity in individuals with epilepsy. Emotional stress, anxiety, and tension can trigger seizures or increase their frequency and severity. Managing stress effectively is essential for optimizing seizure control and improving overall quality of life for individuals with epilepsy.

Stress Reduction Techniques for Epilepsy Management:

1. **Mindfulness Meditation:** Mindfulness meditation involves focusing on the present moment without judgment, allowing individuals to cultivate awareness, acceptance, and inner peace. Regular practice of mindfulness meditation can

reduce stress, promote relaxation, and enhance emotional well-being in individuals with epilepsy.

2. **Deep Breathing Exercises:** Deep breathing exercises, such as diaphragmatic breathing or belly breathing, help activate the body's relaxation response and reduce the physiological effects of stress. Practicing deep breathing techniques regularly can promote calmness, reduce anxiety, and support seizure control.

3. **Progressive Muscle Relaxation:** Progressive muscle relaxation involves systematically tensing and relaxing muscle groups throughout the body, promoting physical and mental relaxation. This technique can help alleviate muscle tension, reduce stress, and improve sleep quality in individuals with epilepsy.

4. **Yoga and Tai Chi:** Yoga and Tai Chi are mind-body practices that combine gentle physical movements with breath awareness and meditation. These practices promote relaxation, flexibility, and balance, while reducing stress and anxiety levels in individuals with epilepsy.

5. **Aromatherapy:** Aromatherapy involves using essential oils derived from aromatic plants to promote relaxation and reduce stress. Inhalation of calming essential oils such as lavender, chamomile, or bergamot can help alleviate anxiety

and support emotional well-being in individuals with epilepsy.

Herbal Support for Stress Reduction and Epilepsy Management:

1. **Lemon Balm (Melissa officinalis):** Lemon balm is prized for its calming and mood-stabilizing effects, making it a valuable herbal remedy for reducing stress and anxiety in individuals with epilepsy.

2. **Passionflower (Passiflora incarnata):** Passionflower has anxiolytic and sedative properties, which can help alleviate stress, promote relaxation, and support seizure control.

3. **Valerian (Valeriana officinalis):** Valerian root is known for its sedative and anxiolytic effects, making it a potential herbal support for reducing stress and anxiety levels in individuals with epilepsy.

4. **Chamomile (Matricaria chamomilla):** Chamomile is prized for its calming and anti-inflammatory properties, which can help reduce stress, promote relaxation, and support overall well-being in individuals with epilepsy.

Incorporating Stress Reduction Techniques and Herbal Support into Your Daily Routine:

1. **Create a Relaxation Ritual:** Set aside time each day for relaxation and stress reduction activities, such as meditation,

deep breathing exercises, or aromatherapy. Establishing a relaxation ritual can help you unwind and manage stress effectively.

2. **Prioritize Self-Care:** Make self-care a priority by engaging in activities that promote physical, mental, and emotional well-being. Practice good sleep hygiene, eat a balanced diet, exercise regularly, and spend time in nature to support overall health and resilience.

3. **Stay Consistent with Herbal Support:** Incorporate herbal remedies known for their stress-reducing properties, such as lemon balm, passionflower, valerian, or chamomile, into your daily routine. Whether as herbal teas, tinctures, or supplements, stay consistent with herbal support for optimal benefits.

4. **Seek Professional Guidance:** Consult with healthcare professionals, including physicians, neurologists, or herbalists, for personalized guidance on stress reduction techniques and herbal support tailored to your individual needs and health goals.

Conclusion:

Stress reduction techniques and herbal support play integral roles in epilepsy management, helping individuals minimize stress, promote relaxation, and optimize seizure control. By incorporating mindfulness practices, deep breathing exercises, aromatherapy, and herbal remedies into your daily routine, you can cultivate resilience, enhance emotional well-being, and support overall health and vitality. Remember to stay consistent with stress reduction techniques and herbal support, seek professional guidance when needed, and prioritize self-care for holistic epilepsy management. Stay tuned for more insights and practical tips on herbal remedies for epilepsy management in the upcoming sessions.

CHAPTER NINE

Day 6: Lifestyle Modifications and Herbal Therapies for Better Seizure Control

Welcome to Day 6 of our series on herbal remedies for epilepsy management. Today, we'll explore lifestyle modifications and herbal therapies aimed at enhancing seizure control and improving overall well-being. By adopting healthy lifestyle practices and incorporating herbal remedies into your daily routine, you can support optimal brain health and minimize seizure frequency and severity. Let's delve into practical strategies for achieving better seizure control through lifestyle changes and herbal therapies.

Lifestyle Modifications for Better Seizure Control:

1. **Maintain a Regular Sleep Schedule:** Prioritize adequate sleep by maintaining a consistent sleep schedule and practicing good sleep hygiene habits. Aim for 7-9 hours of quality sleep each night to support optimal brain function and minimize seizure risk.

2. **Manage Stress Effectively:** Implement stress reduction techniques such as mindfulness meditation, deep breathing exercises, yoga, or aromatherapy to manage stress levels and promote relaxation. Chronic stress can exacerbate

seizure activity, so finding effective stress management strategies is essential.

3. **Stay Hydrated:** Drink plenty of water throughout the day to stay hydrated and support overall health. Dehydration can increase seizure susceptibility, so it's crucial to maintain adequate fluid intake, especially in hot weather or during physical activity.

4. **Eat a Balanced Diet:** Follow a balanced diet rich in fruits, vegetables, whole grains, lean proteins, and healthy fats to provide essential nutrients and support overall well-being. Consider adopting dietary strategies such as the ketogenic diet, which has shown benefits for some individuals with epilepsy.

5. **Exercise Regularly:** Engage in regular physical activity, such as walking, swimming, cycling, or yoga, to promote cardiovascular health, reduce stress, and support overall brain function. Consult with healthcare professionals to determine safe and appropriate exercise options based on your individual health needs.

Herbal Therapies for Better Seizure Control:

1. **Ashwagandha (Withaniasomnifera):** Ashwagandha is an adaptogenic herb known for its stress-relieving and

neuroprotective properties. It may help reduce seizure frequency and promote overall brain health.

2. **Bacopa (Bacopa monnieri):** Bacopa is a cognitive-enhancing herb that may support memory, concentration, and cognitive function in individuals with epilepsy. It has neuroprotective effects and may help reduce seizure severity.

3. **Holy Basil (Ocimum sanctum):** Holy basil, also known as tulsi, is an adaptogenic herb with antioxidant and anti-inflammatory properties. It may help reduce stress, anxiety, and seizure susceptibility.

4. **Ginkgo Biloba (Ginkgo biloba):** Ginkgo biloba extract has neuroprotective effects and may improve cognitive function and reduce seizure frequency in individuals with epilepsy.

5. **Passionflower (Passiflora incarnata):** Passionflower is prized for its calming and sedative effects, making it a valuable herbal remedy for reducing stress, anxiety, and seizure risk.

Incorporating Lifestyle Modifications and Herbal Therapies into Your Routine:

1. **Create a Daily Routine:** Establish a daily routine that incorporates healthy lifestyle practices, stress reduction

techniques, and herbal therapies. Consistency is key to optimizing seizure control and overall well-being.

2. **Set Realistic Goals:** Set realistic goals for implementing lifestyle modifications and herbal therapies into your routine. Start with small changes and gradually incorporate additional practices over time.

3. **Track Your Progress:** Keep track of your seizure frequency, severity, and other relevant symptoms to monitor the effectiveness of lifestyle modifications and herbal therapies. Use a seizure diary or tracking app to record observations and identify patterns.

4. **Stay Informed:** Stay informed about the latest research and developments in epilepsy management, including lifestyle interventions and herbal therapies. Consult with healthcare professionals for personalized guidance and recommendations based on your individual health needs.

5. **Seek Support:** Reach out to support groups, online communities, or healthcare professionals for support, guidance, and encouragement on your journey to better seizure control and overall well-being.

Conclusion:

Lifestyle modifications and herbal therapies offer valuable tools for individuals seeking better seizure control and improved quality of life. By adopting healthy lifestyle practices, managing stress effectively, and incorporating herbal remedies into your routine, you can support optimal brain health, minimize seizure frequency and severity, and enhance overall well-being. Remember to consult with healthcare professionals for personalized guidance and recommendations tailored to your individual health needs. Stay tuned for more insights and practical tips on herbal remedies for epilepsy management in the upcoming sessions.

CHAPTER TEN

Day 7: Monitoring Progress and Planning Continued Herbal Treatment

Welcome to Day 7, the final session of our series on herbal remedies for epilepsy management. Today, we'll focus on monitoring progress and planning continued herbal treatment to ensure long-term success in seizure control and overall well-being. Effective monitoring allows individuals to track their response to herbal therapy, identify any changes in seizure activity, and make informed decisions about ongoing treatment. Let's explore practical strategies for monitoring progress and planning continued herbal treatment for epilepsy management.

Monitoring Progress in Seizure Control:

1. **Keep a Seizure Diary:** Maintain a seizure diary to track the frequency, duration, and severity of seizures over time. Record details such as triggers, aura, postictal symptoms, and any notable changes in seizure patterns. A seizure diary provides valuable insights into your seizure activity and helps identify trends or patterns that may influence treatment decisions.

2. **Use a Symptom Tracker:** In addition to seizures, track other symptoms and related factors such as mood changes, stress

levels, medication side effects, sleep quality, and overall well-being. A symptom tracker can help you assess the impact of herbal therapy on various aspects of your health and identify areas for improvement.

3. **Regular Follow-Up with Healthcare Professionals:** Schedule regular follow-up appointments with healthcare professionals, including physicians, neurologists, or herbalists, to review your progress, discuss any concerns or changes in symptoms, and adjust treatment as needed. Open communication with healthcare providers is essential for optimizing seizure control and overall health.

4. **Objective Assessments:** Consider objective assessments such as electroencephalography (EEG) or imaging studies to evaluate brain activity and identify any underlying abnormalities or changes in response to herbal therapy. These assessments can provide valuable information about treatment efficacy and guide treatment decisions.

Planning Continued Herbal Treatment:

1. **Review Treatment Goals:** Review your treatment goals and objectives in collaboration with healthcare professionals. Assess whether your current herbal therapy regimen aligns with your goals for seizure control, overall well-being, and quality of life.

2. **Adjust Dosage or Formulation:** Based on your progress and feedback, healthcare professionals may recommend adjusting the dosage, formulation, or combination of herbal remedies to optimize treatment outcomes. Individualize treatment based on your response to herbal therapy and any changes in seizure activity or related symptoms.

3. **Explore Complementary Therapies:** Consider integrating complementary therapies such as acupuncture, chiropractic care, or dietary supplements into your epilepsy management plan to enhance overall health and well-being. Collaborate with healthcare professionals to explore safe and evidence-based complementary approaches.

4. **Stay Informed and Educated:** Stay informed about the latest research, developments, and emerging trends in herbal medicine and epilepsy management. Attend educational events, workshops, or support groups to expand your knowledge and empower yourself with information to make informed decisions about your health.

5. **Maintain Lifestyle Modifications:** Continue practicing healthy lifestyle habits, stress reduction techniques, and other supportive measures alongside herbal therapy to maximize seizure control and overall well-being. Consistency is key to long-term success in epilepsy management.

Conclusion:

Monitoring progress and planning continued herbal treatment are essential components of a comprehensive approach to epilepsy management. By keeping track of seizure activity, symptoms, and treatment response, individuals can make informed decisions about ongoing herbal therapy, optimize treatment outcomes, and enhance overall quality of life. Collaborating with healthcare professionals, staying informed, and maintaining a holistic approach to health and wellness are key to long-term success in managing epilepsy with herbal remedies. Remember that individual responses to herbal therapy may vary, and it's essential to work closely with healthcare professionals to tailor treatment to your specific needs and goals. Thank you for joining us in this series, and we wish you success and well-being on your journey to optimal seizure control and overall health.

BONUS: SOME VITAL HERBAL AND NATURAL REMEDIES YOU SHOULD KNOW

Hydrangea:

Definition: Hydrangea, scientifically known as Hydrangea arborescens, is a flowering shrub native to North America. It has been used traditionally in herbal medicine for its potential diuretic and anti-inflammatory properties.

Ingredients: Hydrangea contains several bioactive compounds, including saponins, flavonoids, and glycosides. These compounds are believed to contribute to the herb's medicinal properties, including its potential as a diuretic, kidney tonic, and anti-inflammatory agent.

How to Prepare: Hydrangea root is typically prepared and consumed as an herbal tea or tincture. To make tea, dried hydrangea root is steeped in hot water for several minutes before being strained and consumed. Tinctures are prepared by steeping the root in alcohol or vinegar to extract its active compounds.

Dosage: The appropriate dosage of hydrangea can vary depending on factors such as age, health status, and the specific preparation being used. It's important to follow the recommended dosage on the product label or consult with a qualified herbalist or healthcare professional for personalized guidance.

How to Use: Hydrangea tea or tincture is typically taken orally. It's important to use hydrangea products as directed and to discontinue use if any adverse effects occur.

Side Effects: Hydrangea is generally considered safe for most people when used in moderate amounts. However, some individuals may experience digestive upset or allergic reactions. It may also interact with certain medications or have adverse effects in individuals with certain health conditions. It's important to use hydrangea under the guidance of a healthcare professional and to discontinue use if any adverse effects occur.

Irish Moss:

Definition: Irish Moss, scientifically known as Chondrus crispus, is a species of red algae or seaweed native to the Atlantic coastlines of Europe and North America. It has been used for centuries in traditional Irish and Scottish cuisine, as well as in herbal medicine.

Ingredients: Irish Moss is rich in various nutrients, including iodine, sulfur compounds, vitamins (such as vitamin A, vitamin K, and vitamin B12), minerals (including calcium, magnesium, potassium, and sodium), and polysaccharides (such as carrageenan). These nutrients are believed to contribute to the herb's potential health benefits.

How to Prepare: Irish Moss is typically prepared by soaking it in water to rehydrate and soften it before use. It can be added to soups, stews, smoothies, desserts, and other dishes as a thickening agent or nutritional supplement.

Dosage: The appropriate dosage of Irish Moss can vary depending on factors such as age, health status, and the specific preparation being used. It's important to follow recipes or guidelines for culinary use and to consult with a healthcare professional for guidance on using Irish Moss as a dietary supplement.

How to Use: Irish Moss can be used in culinary applications to add thickness and nutritional value to dishes. It can also be consumed as a dietary supplement in the form of capsules, powders, or extracts.

Side Effects: Irish Moss is generally considered safe for most people when consumed in moderate amounts as part of a balanced diet. However, some individuals may be allergic to seaweed or carrageenan, a compound found in Irish Moss that is used as a food additive. It's important to discontinue use if any adverse effects occur and to consult with a healthcare professional if you have any concerns.

Irish Sea Moss:

Definition: Irish Sea Moss is a term often used interchangeably with Irish Moss, referring to the same species of red algae, Chondrus crispus. It's harvested from the rocky shores of the Atlantic coastlines of Europe and North America.

Ingredients: Irish Sea Moss shares the same nutritional profile as Irish Moss, containing iodine, vitamins, minerals, and polysaccharides. It's valued for its potential health benefits, including supporting thyroid function, boosting immune health, and promoting digestion.

How to Prepare: Irish Sea Moss is prepared in the same way as Irish Moss, by soaking it in water to rehydrate and soften it before use. It can be used in culinary applications or consumed as a dietary supplement.

Dosage: The dosage of Irish Sea Moss depends on the form and intended use. As a dietary supplement, it's important to follow the recommended dosage on the product label or consult with a healthcare professional for personalized guidance.

How to Use: Irish Sea Moss can be used in various culinary applications, including soups, smoothies, desserts, and sauces. It can also be consumed as a dietary supplement in the form of capsules, powders, or extracts.

Side Effects: Similar to Irish Moss, Irish Sea Moss is generally considered safe for most people when consumed in moderate amounts. However, individuals with seaweed allergies or sensitivities to carrageenan should exercise caution. It's important to discontinue use if any adverse effects occur and to consult with a healthcare professional if you have any concerns.

Lymphalin:

Definition: Lymphalin is a herbal supplement formulated to support lymphatic system health. The lymphatic system plays a crucial role in immune function and waste removal in the body, and Lymphalin is designed to promote its proper function.

Ingredients: Lymphalin typically contains a blend of herbs and botanical extracts known for their traditional use in supporting lymphatic system health. Common ingredients may include cleavers, red clover, echinacea, burdock root, and calendula, among others.

How to Prepare: Lymphalin is usually available in capsule or liquid form. Capsules are taken orally with water, while liquid forms may be mixed with water or juice before consumption. It's important to follow the recommended dosage on the product label.

Dosage: The appropriate dosage of Lymphalin can vary depending on the specific product and individual needs. It's important to follow the recommended dosage on the product label or consult with a healthcare professional for personalized guidance.

How to Use: Lymphalin capsules are typically taken orally with water, while liquid forms may be mixed with water or juice before consumption. It's often recommended to take Lymphalin on an empty stomach for optimal absorption.

Side Effects: Lymphalin is generally considered safe for most people when used as directed. However, some individuals may experience mild side effects such as gastrointestinal discomfort or allergic reactions to certain ingredients. It's important to consult with a healthcare provider before starting any new supplement regimen, especially if you have underlying health conditions or are taking medications.

Manjakani:

Definition: Manjakani, also known as Quercus infectoria or oak gall, is a natural substance derived from the oak tree. It has been used for centuries in traditional medicine for its potential health benefits, particularly for women's health and vaginal tightening.

Ingredients: Manjakani contains various bioactive compounds, including tannins, flavonoids, and gallic acid. These compounds are believed to contribute to the herb's medicinal properties, including its potential as an astringent and antiseptic agent.

How to Prepare: Manjakani is typically available in powder, capsule, or liquid extract form. It can be taken orally or used topically depending on the intended use. For vaginal tightening, manjakani may be applied topically as a gel or inserted into the vagina in capsule form.

Dosage: The appropriate dosage of manjakani can vary depending on factors such as age, health status, and the specific preparation being used. It's important to follow the recommended dosage on the product label or consult with a qualified herbalist or healthcare professional for personalized guidance.

How to Use: Manjakani can be taken orally or used topically depending on the intended use. It's important to use manjakani products as directed and to discontinue use if any adverse effects occur.

Side Effects: Manjakani is generally considered safe for most people when used in moderate amounts. However, some individuals may experience allergic reactions or skin irritation when used topically. It's important to use manjakani under the guidance of a healthcare professional and to discontinue use if any adverse effects occur.

Red Clover:

Definition: Red clover, scientifically known as Trifolium pratense, is a flowering plant belonging to the legume family. It's native to Europe, Western Asia, and Northwest Africa but has been naturalized in many other regions. Red clover has been used in traditional medicine for various purposes, including its potential to support women's health and menopausal symptoms.

Ingredients: Red clover contains several bioactive compounds, including isoflavones (such as genistein and daidzein), flavonoids, and phytoestrogens. These compounds are believed to contribute to the herb's medicinal properties, including its potential as a hormone-balancing agent and its ability to support cardiovascular health.

How to Prepare: Red clover is typically prepared and consumed as an herbal tea or tincture. To make tea, dried red clover flowers are steeped in hot water for several minutes before being strained and consumed. Tinctures are prepared by steeping the flowers in alcohol or vinegar to extract their active compounds.

Dosage: The appropriate dosage of red clover can vary depending on factors such as age, health status, and the specific preparation being used. It's important to follow the recommended dosage on the product label or consult with a qualified herbalist or healthcare professional for personalized guidance.

How to Use: Red clover tea or tincture is typically taken orally. It's important to use red clover products as directed and to discontinue use if any adverse effects occur.

Side Effects: Red clover is generally considered safe for most people when used in moderate amounts. However, some individuals may experience allergic reactions or digestive upset. It may also interact with certain medications or have adverse effects in individuals with certain health conditions. It's important to use red clover under the guidance of a healthcare professional and to discontinue use if any adverse effects occur.

Red Raspberry:

Definition: Red raspberry, scientifically known as Rubus idaeus, is a species of raspberry native to Europe and northern Asia. It's widely cultivated for its delicious berries and has been used in traditional medicine for various purposes, including its potential to support women's health during pregnancy and childbirth.

Ingredients: Red raspberry contains several bioactive compounds, including flavonoids, ellagic acid, anthocyanins, and vitamin C. These compounds are believed to contribute to the herb's medicinal properties, including its potential as an antioxidant, anti-inflammatory, and uterine tonic.

How to Prepare: Red raspberry leaf is typically prepared and consumed as an herbal tea or infusion. To make tea, dried red raspberry leaves are steeped in hot water for several minutes before being strained and consumed.

Dosage: The appropriate dosage of red raspberry leaf can vary depending on factors such as age, health status, and the specific preparation being used. It's important to follow the recommended dosage on the product label or consult with a qualified herbalist or healthcare professional for personalized guidance.

How to Use: Red raspberry leaf tea is typically taken orally. It's often recommended for pregnant individuals in the later stages of pregnancy to support uterine health and prepare for childbirth. It's important to use red raspberry leaf products as directed and to discontinue use if any adverse effects occur.

Side Effects: Red raspberry leaf is generally considered safe for most people when used in moderate amounts. However, some individuals may experience allergic reactions or digestive upset. Pregnant individuals should consult with a healthcare professional before using red raspberry leaf, especially if they have any underlying health conditions or are taking medications. It's important to use red raspberry leaf under the guidance of a healthcare professional and to discontinue use if any adverse effects occur.

Rhubarb:

Definition: Rhubarb, scientifically known as Rheum rhabarbarum, is a perennial plant cultivated for its edible stalks. While primarily used in culinary applications, rhubarb has also been utilized in traditional medicine for its potential health benefits, particularly for digestive health.

Ingredients: Rhubarb stalks contain various bioactive compounds, including anthraquinones (such as emodin and rhein), fiber, vitamins (such as vitamin K), and minerals (including calcium and potassium). These compounds are believed to contribute to the herb's medicinal properties, including its potential as a laxative and digestive aid.

How to Prepare: Rhubarb stalks are typically cooked before consumption, as the raw stalks are very tart and can be unpleasant to eat. They are often used in pies, crisps, jams, sauces, and other desserts, as well as in savory dishes. Rhubarb can also be used to make compotes, jams, and preserves.

Dosage: There is no specific dosage for rhubarb in culinary applications, as it is used as a food rather than a medicinal herb. However, when used for its potential laxative effects, it's important to consume rhubarb in moderation to avoid gastrointestinal upset.

How to Use: Rhubarb stalks can be chopped and cooked in various dishes, including pies, sauces, and jams. It's important to remove and discard the leaves, as they contain toxic compounds. When using rhubarb for its potential laxative effects, it's typically consumed as part of a cooked dish or in the form of a rhubarb-based herbal remedy.

Side Effects: Rhubarb stalks are generally safe for most people when consumed in moderate amounts as part of a balanced diet. However, excessive intake may lead to digestive upset or adverse effects due to the presence of oxalic acid, which can bind to calcium and form kidney stones in susceptible individuals. It's important to use rhubarb in moderation and to consult with a healthcare professional if you have any concerns or underlying health conditions.

Sarsaparilla:

Definition: Sarsaparilla refers to several species of plants belonging to the Smilax genus, including Smilax regelii and Smilax officinalis. It has been used historically in traditional medicine for its potential health benefits, particularly for its purported detoxifying and anti-inflammatory properties.

Ingredients: Sarsaparilla contains various bioactive compounds, including saponins (such as sarsaponin and smilagenin), flavonoids, phenolic acids, and sterols. These compounds are believed to contribute to the herb's medicinal properties, including its potential as a diuretic, blood purifier, and anti-inflammatory agent.

How to Prepare: Sarsaparilla root is typically prepared and consumed as an herbal tea, decoction, or tincture. To make tea, dried sarsaparilla root is steeped in hot water for several minutes before being strained and consumed. Decoctions involve boiling the root in water to extract its active compounds, while tinctures are prepared by steeping the root in alcohol or vinegar.

Dosage: The appropriate dosage of sarsaparilla can vary depending on factors such as age, health status, and the specific preparation being used. It's important to follow the recommended dosage on the product label or consult with a qualified herbalist or healthcare professional for personalized guidance.

How to Use: Sarsaparilla tea or tincture is typically taken orally. It's important to use sarsaparilla products as directed and to discontinue use if any adverse effects occur.

Side Effects: Sarsaparilla is generally considered safe for most people when used in moderate amounts. However, some individuals may experience allergic reactions or digestive upset. It may also interact with certain medications or have adverse effects in individuals with certain health conditions. It's important to use sarsaparilla under the guidance of a healthcare professional and to discontinue use if any adverse effects occur.

Tila:

Definition: Tila, also known as linden flower or lime blossom, refers to the flowers of the Tilia genus, primarily Tilia europaea and Tilia cordata. These trees are native to Europe, but they are also cultivated in other regions for their fragrant and medicinal flowers.

Ingredients: Tila flowers contain various bioactive compounds, including flavonoids, phenolic acids, and volatile oils. These compounds are believed to contribute to the herb's medicinal properties, including its potential as a mild sedative, anxiolytic, and anti-inflammatory agent.

How to Prepare: Tila flowers are typically prepared and consumed as an herbal tea or infusion. To make tea, dried tila flowers are steeped in hot water for several minutes before being strained and consumed.

Dosage: The appropriate dosage of tila can vary depending on factors such as age, health status, and the specific preparation being used. It's important to follow the recommended dosage on the product label or consult with a qualified herbalist or healthcare professional for personalized guidance.

How to Use: Tila tea is typically taken orally. It's often consumed in the evening as a calming bedtime beverage or during times of stress or anxiety. It's important to use tila products as directed and to discontinue use if any adverse effects occur.

Side Effects: Tila is generally considered safe for most people when used in moderate amounts. However, some individuals may experience allergic reactions or digestive upset. It may also interact with certain medications or have adverse effects in individuals with certain health conditions. It's important to use tila under the guidance of a healthcare professional and to discontinue use if any adverse effects occur.

Valerian:

Definition: Valerian, scientifically known as Valeriana officinalis, is a perennial flowering plant native to Europe and Asia. It has been used for centuries in traditional medicine for its potential calming and sedative effects.

Ingredients: Valerian root contains several bioactive compounds, including valerenic acid, valepotriates, and volatile oils. These compounds are believed to contribute to the herb's medicinal properties, including its potential as a sedative, anxiolytic, and sleep aid.

How to Prepare: Valerian root is typically prepared and consumed as an herbal tea, tincture, or capsule. To make tea, dried valerian root is steeped in hot water for several minutes before being strained and consumed. Tinctures are prepared by steeping the root in alcohol or vinegar to extract its active compounds.

Dosage: The appropriate dosage of valerian can vary depending on factors such as age, health status, and the specific preparation being used. It's important to follow the recommended dosage on the product label or consult with a qualified herbalist or healthcare professional for personalized guidance.

How to Use: Valerian tea, tincture, or capsules are typically taken orally. It's often consumed in the evening as a sleep aid or during times of stress or anxiety. It's important to use valerian products as directed and to discontinue use if any adverse effects occur.

Side Effects: Valerian is generally considered safe for most people when used in moderate amounts. However, some individuals may experience mild side effects such as drowsiness, headache, or gastrointestinal upset. It may also interact with certain medications or have adverse effects in individuals with certain health conditions. It's important to use valerian under the guidance of a healthcare professional and to discontinue use if any adverse effects occur.

Yellowdock Root:

Definition: Yellowdock root, scientifically known as Rumex crispus, is the root of a perennial flowering plant native to Europe and western Asia, also found in North America. It has a long history of use in traditional medicine, particularly among Indigenous peoples, for its potential health benefits.

Ingredients: Yellowdock root contains various bioactive compounds, including anthraquinone glycosides (such as emodin and chrysophanol), tannins, and vitamins (including vitamin A and vitamin C). These compounds are believed to contribute to the herb's medicinal properties, including its potential as a laxative, blood cleanser, and liver tonic.

How to Prepare: Yellowdock root is typically prepared and consumed as an herbal tea, tincture, or capsule. To make tea, dried yellowdock root is steeped in hot water for several minutes before being strained and consumed. Tinctures are prepared by steeping the root in alcohol or vinegar to extract its active compounds.

Dosage: The appropriate dosage of yellowdock root can vary depending on factors such as age, health status, and the specific preparation being used. It's important to follow the recommended dosage on the product label or consult with a qualified herbalist or healthcare professional for personalized guidance.

How to Use: Yellowdock root tea, tincture, or capsules are typically taken orally. It's often consumed to support digestion, promote bowel regularity, and cleanse the blood. It's important to use yellowdock root products as directed and to discontinue use if any adverse effects occur.

Side Effects: Yellowdock root is generally considered safe for most people when used in moderate amounts. However, some individuals may experience mild side effects such as gastrointestinal upset or allergic reactions. It may also interact with certain medications or have adverse effects in individuals with certain health conditions. It's important to use yellowdock root under the guidance of a healthcare professional and to discontinue use if any adverse effects occur.

Agrimony:

Definition: Agrimony, scientifically known as Agrimonia eupatoria, is a perennial herbaceous plant native to Europe, Asia, and North America. It has a long history of use in traditional medicine, particularly in European folk medicine, for its potential health benefits.

Ingredients: Agrimony contains various bioactive compounds, including tannins, flavonoids, phenolic acids, and volatile oils. These compounds are believed to contribute to the herb's medicinal properties, including its potential as an astringent, anti-inflammatory, and digestive aid.

How to Prepare: Agrimony is typically prepared and consumed as an herbal tea, tincture, or poultice. To make tea, dried agrimony leaves and flowers are steeped in hot water for several minutes before being strained and consumed. Tinctures are prepared by steeping the herb in alcohol or vinegar to extract its active compounds.

Dosage: The appropriate dosage of agrimony can vary depending on factors such as age, health status, and the specific preparation being used. It's important to follow the recommended dosage on the product label or consult with a qualified herbalist or healthcare professional for personalized guidance.

How to Use: Agrimony tea, tincture, or poultice is typically taken orally or applied topically. It's often consumed to soothe gastrointestinal issues, such as indigestion and diarrhea, or used externally to treat skin conditions.

Side Effects: Agrimony is generally considered safe for most people when used in moderate amounts. However, some individuals may experience allergic reactions or gastrointestinal upset. It may also interact with certain medications or have adverse effects in individuals with certain health conditions. It's important to use agrimony under the guidance of a healthcare professional and to discontinue use if any adverse effects occur.

Alfalfa:

Definition: Alfalfa, scientifically known as Medicago sativa, is a flowering plant in the pea family native to Asia but cultivated worldwide. It's primarily grown as fodder for livestock, but it has also been used in traditional medicine for its potential health benefits.

Ingredients: Alfalfa contains various bioactive compounds, including vitamins (such as vitamin A, vitamin C, and vitamin K), minerals (including calcium, magnesium, and potassium), amino acids, and phytoestrogens. These compounds are believed to contribute to the herb's medicinal properties, including its potential as a nutritive tonic, diuretic, and hormone balancer.

How to Prepare: Alfalfa is typically consumed as sprouts, herbal tea, or in supplement form (such as capsules or tablets). To make tea, dried alfalfa leaves are steeped in hot water for several minutes before being strained and consumed.

Dosage: The appropriate dosage of alfalfa can vary depending on factors such as age, health status, and the specific preparation being used. It's important to follow the recommended dosage on the product label or consult with a qualified herbalist or healthcare professional for personalized guidance.

How to Use: Alfalfa sprouts, tea, or supplements are typically taken orally. It's often consumed as a dietary supplement to support overall health and well-being, as well as to promote kidney health and hormone balance.

Side Effects: Alfalfa is generally considered safe for most people when consumed in moderate amounts. However, some individuals may experience allergic reactions or digestive upset. It may also interact with certain medications or have adverse effects in individuals with certain health conditions, such as autoimmune diseases or hormone-sensitive conditions. Pregnant or breastfeeding individuals should consult with a healthcare professional before using alfalfa supplements. It's important to use alfalfa under the guidance of a healthcare professional and to discontinue use if any adverse effects occur.

Ashwagandha:

Definition: Ashwagandha, scientifically known as Withaniasomnifera, is a small shrub native to India, the Middle East, and parts of Africa. It has a long history of use in Ayurvedic medicine for its potential health benefits, particularly for its adaptogenic properties.

Ingredients: Ashwagandha root contains various bioactive compounds, including alkaloids (such as withanolides), steroidal lactones, and flavonoids. These compounds are believed to contribute to the herb's medicinal properties, including its potential as an adaptogen, anti-inflammatory, and immune-modulating agent.

How to Prepare: Ashwagandha is typically consumed as a powdered root, herbal tea, tincture, or in supplement form (such as capsules or tablets). To make tea, dried ashwagandha root is steeped in hot water for several minutes before being strained and consumed.

Dosage: The appropriate dosage of ashwagandha can vary depending on factors such as age, health status, and the specific preparation being used. It's important to follow the recommended dosage on the product label or consult with a qualified herbalist or healthcare professional for personalized guidance.

How to Use: Ashwagandha powder, tea, tincture, or supplements are typically taken orally. It's often consumed to support stress management, promote relaxation, and boost overall vitality and well-being.

Side Effects: Ashwagandha is generally considered safe for most people when used in moderate amounts. However, some individuals may experience mild side effects such as gastrointestinal upset or drowsiness. It may also interact with certain medications or have adverse effects in individuals with certain health conditions, such as autoimmune diseases or thyroid disorders. Pregnant or breastfeeding individuals should consult with a healthcare professional before using ashwagandha supplements. It's important to use ashwagandha under the guidance of a healthcare professional and to discontinue use if any adverse effects occur.

Astragalus:

Definition: Astragalus, scientifically known as Astragalus membranaceus, is a flowering plant native to China and Mongolia but also found in other parts of Asia. It has been used for centuries in traditional Chinese medicine for its potential health benefits, particularly for its immune-enhancing properties.

Ingredients: Astragalus root contains various bioactive compounds, including polysaccharides, saponins (such as astragalosides), flavonoids, and amino acids. These compounds are believed to contribute to the herb's medicinal properties, including its potential as an adaptogen, immunomodulator, and anti-inflammatory agent.

How to Prepare: Astragalus is typically consumed as a powdered root, herbal tea, tincture, or in supplement form (such as capsules or tablets). To make tea, dried astragalus root slices are simmered in water for several minutes before being strained and consumed.

Dosage: The appropriate dosage of astragalus can vary depending on factors such as age, health status, and the specific preparation being used. It's important to follow the recommended dosage on the product label or consult with a qualified herbalist or healthcare professional for personalized guidance.

How to Use: Astragalus powder, tea, tincture, or supplements are typically taken orally. It's often consumed to support immune function, promote vitality, and enhance overall well-being.

Side Effects: Astragalus is generally considered safe for most people when used in moderate amounts. However, some individuals may experience mild side effects such as gastrointestinal upset or allergic reactions. It may also interact with certain medications or have adverse effects in individuals with certain health conditions, such as autoimmune diseases or diabetes. Pregnant or breastfeeding individuals should consult with a healthcare professional before using astragalus supplements. It's important to use astragalus under the guidance of a healthcare professional and to discontinue use if any adverse effects occur.

Black Cohosh:

Definition: Black cohosh, scientifically known as Actaea racemosa (formerly Cimicifuga racemosa), is a perennial herb native to North America. It has a long history of use in traditional Native American medicine and later in folk medicine for its potential health benefits, particularly for women's health.

Ingredients: Black cohosh root contains various bioactive compounds, including triterpene glycosides (such as actein and cimicifugoside), phenolic acids, and flavonoids. These compounds are believed to contribute to the herb's medicinal properties, including its potential as a hormone-balancing agent and its ability to relieve menopausal symptoms.

How to Prepare: Black cohosh is typically consumed as a powdered root, herbal tea, tincture, or in supplement form (such as capsules or tablets). To make tea, dried black cohosh root is steeped in hot water for several minutes before being strained and consumed.

Dosage: The appropriate dosage of black cohosh can vary depending on factors such as age, health status, and the specific preparation being used. It's important to follow the recommended dosage on the product label or consult with a qualified herbalist or healthcare professional for personalized guidance.

How to Use: Black cohosh powder, tea, tincture, or supplements are typically taken orally. It's often used by women to support hormonal balance, relieve menopausal symptoms such as hot flashes and night sweats, and promote overall well-being.

Side Effects: Black cohosh is generally considered safe for most people when used in moderate amounts. However, some individuals may experience mild side effects such as gastrointestinal upset or allergic reactions. It may also interact with certain medications or have adverse effects in individuals with certain health conditions, such as liver disease or hormone-sensitive conditions. Pregnant or breastfeeding individuals should consult with a healthcare professional before using black cohosh supplements. It's important to use black cohosh under the guidance of a healthcare professional and to discontinue use if any adverse effects occur.

Wild Cherry Bark:

Definition: Wild cherry bark, scientifically known as Prunus serotina, is the bark obtained from the black cherry tree native to North America. It has been used traditionally in Native American and folk medicine for its potential health benefits, particularly for respiratory and digestive issues.

Ingredients: Wild cherry bark contains various bioactive compounds, including cyanogenic glycosides (such as prunasin and amygdalin), flavonoids, and phenolic acids. These compounds are believed to contribute to the herb's medicinal properties, including its potential as an expectorant, cough suppressant, and mild sedative.

How to Prepare: Wild cherry bark is typically prepared and consumed as an herbal tea, decoction, or syrup. To make tea, dried wild cherry bark is steeped in hot water for several minutes before being strained and consumed. Decoctions involve boiling the bark in water to extract its active compounds, while syrups are made by simmering the bark with sugar or honey to create a thick, sweet liquid.

Dosage: The appropriate dosage of wild cherry bark can vary depending on factors such as age, health status, and the specific preparation being used. It's important to follow the recommended dosage on the product label or consult with a qualified herbalist or healthcare professional for personalized guidance.

How to Use: Wild cherry bark tea, decoction, or syrup is typically taken orally. It's often consumed to soothe coughs, sore throats, and other respiratory symptoms. It's important to use wild cherry bark products as directed and to discontinue use if any adverse effects occur.

Side Effects: Wild cherry bark is generally considered safe for most people when used in moderate amounts. However, it contains cyanogenic glycosides, which can release cyanide in the body when metabolized. While the risk of cyanide poisoning from consuming wild cherry bark is low when used appropriately, excessive intake or prolonged use may lead to adverse effects. It's important to use wild cherry bark under the guidance of a healthcare professional and to discontinue use if any adverse effects occur.

Yellowdock:

Definition: Yellowdock, scientifically known as Rumex crispus, is a perennial flowering plant native to Europe and western Asia but is also found in North America. It has a long history of use in traditional medicine, particularly among Indigenous peoples, for its potential health benefits.

Ingredients: Yellowdock root contains various bioactive compounds, including anthraquinone glycosides (such as emodin and chrysophanol), tannins, and vitamins (including vitamin A and vitamin C). These compounds are believed to contribute to the herb's medicinal properties, including its potential as a laxative, blood cleanser, and liver tonic.

How to Prepare: Yellowdock root is typically prepared and consumed as an herbal tea, tincture, or capsule. To make tea, dried yellowdock root is steeped in hot water for several minutes before being strained and consumed. Tinctures are prepared by steeping the root in alcohol or vinegar to extract its active compounds.

Dosage: The appropriate dosage of yellowdock can vary depending on factors such as age, health status, and the specific preparation being used. It's important to follow the recommended dosage on the product label or consult with a qualified herbalist or healthcare professional for personalized guidance.

How to Use: Yellowdock tea, tincture, or capsules are typically taken orally. It's often consumed to support digestion, promote bowel regularity, and cleanse the blood. It's important to use yellowdock products as directed and to discontinue use if any adverse effects occur.

Side Effects: Yellowdock is generally considered safe for most people when used in moderate amounts. However, some individuals may experience mild side effects such as gastrointestinal upset or allergic reactions. It may also interact with certain medications or have adverse effects in individuals with certain health conditions. It's important to use yellowdock under the guidance of a healthcare professional and to discontinue use if any adverse effects occur.

THE END